Osteoarthritis chronicles

A comprehensive guide to maintaining a healthy joint and bones

Dr lawson davies

Copyright

No part of this book should be copied replaced or
printed out without authors permission

TABLE OF CONTENT

Introduction

Osteoarthritis (OA) is a common and debilitating joint disorder that primarily affects the elderly but can also occur in younger individuals due to various factors. It is the most prevalent form of arthritis, characterized by the progressive degradation of joint cartilage and the underlying bone. While OA can affect any joint, it most frequently impacts the knees, hips, hands, and spine.

The main causes of OA include aging, genetics, obesity, joint overuse or trauma, and underlying joint abnormalities. As people age, the cartilage that cushions their joints begins to break down, leading to pain, swelling, and limited mobility. Genetic factors can predispose individuals to OA, making it more likely for the disease to develop in their joints.

Obesity is a significant risk factor for OA, especially in weight-bearing joints like the knees and hips, as the extra weight places increased stress on these joints. Joint overuse or trauma, such as sports injuries or accidents, can also accelerate the development of OA by damaging the joint structures. Additionally, preexisting joint abnormalities can make one more susceptible to the condition.

Symptoms of OA include joint pain, stiffness, and reduced range of motion, which can have a significant impact on an individual's quality of life. While there is no cure for OA, various treatment options aim to alleviate symptoms and improve joint function. These may include lifestyle modifications, such as weight management and exercise, as well as medications to manage pain and inflammation. In severe cases, joint replacement surgery may be necessary to restore mobility and reduce pain.

Overall, osteoarthritis is a chronic and progressive condition that can have a
profound impact on an individual's well-being. Early diagnosis and management are key to minimizing its effects and improving the quality of life for those living with this condition. Researchers continue to explore new therapies and interventions to better understand and treat OA, with the hope of providing more effective solutions in the future.

Chapter 1

Introduction to Osteoarthritis

Osteoarthritis is a prevalent and degenerative joint disease that affects millions of people worldwide, primarily in the aging population. It is a chronic condition characterized by the gradual breakdown of joint cartilage, which serves as a cushion and lubricant for the bones, causing pain, stiffness, and reduced joint mobility. While the exact cause of osteoarthritis remains elusive, it is believed to result from a combination of genetic, mechanical, and environmental factors.

The hallmark of osteoarthritis is the erosion of the protective cartilage, leading to bone-on-bone contact, inflammation, and the formation of bone spurs. This process can affect any joint but commonly occurs in weight-bearing joints like the knees, hips, and spine. Over time, osteoarthritis can have a significant impact on an individual's quality of life, as it limits their ability to perform everyday activities and may lead to disability.

Diagnosis typically involves a clinical assessment, X-rays, and sometimes MRI scans to evaluate joint damage. While there is no cure for osteoarthritis, various treatment options exist to manage symptoms and improve joint function. These may include lifestyle modifications, physical therapy, pain relievers, and in severe cases, surgical interventions such as joint replacement surgery.

Understanding osteoarthritis is crucial for both patients and healthcare providers, as early intervention and management can significantly alleviate its impact and improve the overall well-being of those affected by this common joint ailment.

.

Definition and Overview

Osteoarthritis is a prevalent joint condition characterized by the gradual deterioration of cartilage, the protective tissue that cushions and lubricates the joints. This degenerative disease commonly affects weight-bearing joints like the knees, hips, and spine, leading to symptoms such as pain, stiffness, and reduced mobility. Osteoarthritis primarily afflicts the aging population, but it can also result from joint injuries, genetics, and obesity. As cartilage wears away, bone-on-bone contact, inflammation, and the development of bone spurs occur. While there is no cure for osteoarthritis, treatment options focus on managing symptoms and may involve lifestyle changes, physical therapy, pain relief medications, and, in severe cases, surgical interventions.

Prevalence and Incidence

Osteoarthritis is a highly prevalent joint disorder that places a significant burden on global healthcare systems. Its prevalence and incidence are influenced by a multitude of factors, making it a widespread and growing concern.

The prevalence of osteoarthritis varies with age, and it primarily affects the elderly population. As people age, the risk of developing osteoarthritis increases. It's estimated that nearly 27 million Americans are affected by osteoarthritis, with higher rates among women. Additionally, the rising rates of obesity contribute to the increased prevalence of osteoarthritis, as excess body weight places additional stress on weight-bearing joints.

The incidence of osteoarthritis is also influenced by factors such as genetics, joint injuries, and occupational activities. Sports-related injuries, repetitive movements, and jobs that involve heavy lifting or prolonged standing can raise the risk of developing this condition. As a result, the incidence of osteoarthritis is rising, particularly among younger individuals.

With the global aging population and lifestyle changes, the prevalence and incidence of osteoarthritis are expected to continue to rise in the coming years. This poses a substantial public health challenge, necessitating proactive measures for prevention, early diagnosis, and effective management to alleviate the pain and disability associated with this common joint disorder.

Historical Perspective

Osteoarthritis has a long historical perspective, with evidence of its presence dating back thousands of years. Understanding its historical context provides insights into the evolution of our knowledge and treatment of this joint disorder.

Ancient Egyptian and Greek medical texts mention joint-related conditions that could be early references to osteoarthritis. Hippocrates, the ancient Greek physician, described a condition similar to osteoarthritis in his writings, referring to joint pain and stiffness.

In the Middle Ages, osteoarthritis was often associated with aging, and its management focused on herbal remedies and dietary changes. It was considered a natural consequence of growing older.

It wasn't until the 18th and 19th centuries that more systematic observations and studies on osteoarthritis began to emerge. French surgeon Jean-Martin Charcot made significant contributions to our understanding of joint diseases, including osteoarthritis. The term "osteoarthritis" itself was coined in the 1850s.

Advancements in medical imaging and research in the 20th century allowed for a deeper understanding of the pathophysiology of osteoarthritis. This period saw the development of joint replacement surgeries, which revolutionized the treatment of advanced cases.

Today, our historical perspective on osteoarthritis has paved the way for a comprehensive understanding of the disease, leading to a range of treatment options, from lifestyle modifications to surgical interventions. Ongoing research continues to enhance our knowledge and improve the quality of life for individuals affected by this common joint ailment.

Joint structure and function

Osteoarthritis (OA) is a degenerative joint disorder that primarily affects the structure and function of synovial joints, such as the knees, hips, and hands. Understanding the interplay between joint structure and function in OA is crucial for managing this common age-related condition.

The joint structure is a complex system consisting of several key components. Articular cartilage, which covers the ends of bones, plays a pivotal role. In OA, this cartilage begins to deteriorate, leading to increased friction and damage within the joint. As cartilage wears away, the underlying bone may develop bony growths called osteophytes, further disrupting joint function.

The synovial membrane, which produces synovial fluid, lubricates the joint and nourishes the cartilage. In OA, inflammation of the synovial membrane can lead to increased production of synovial fluid, contributing to joint swelling and pain.

As joint structure deteriorates, joint function is compromised. Patients with OA experience pain, stiffness, and reduced mobility. Activities of daily living become challenging, and the joint's range of motion diminishes.

Management of OA focuses on alleviating symptoms, preserving joint function, and enhancing the patient's quality of life. Non-pharmacological interventions like physical therapy, weight management, and assistive devices are crucial. Medications, such as pain relievers and anti-inflammatory drugs, can be prescribed. In severe cases, surgical interventions like joint replacement may be necessary.

Understanding the intricate relationship between joint structure and function in osteoarthritis is vital for providing effective care and improving the lives of those affected by this prevalent musculoskeletal condition.

Chapter 2

Osteoarthritis is a complex condition with multifactorial causes and risk factors that contribute to its development. Understanding these factors is crucial for prevention and management.

1. Age: Increasing age is a primary risk factor for osteoarthritis. The natural wear and tear of joints over time make older individuals more susceptible to the condition.

2. Genetics: Family history plays a role, as genetics can influence the development of osteoarthritis. Some people may inherit genes that make them more prone to joint problems.

3. Joint Injuries: Past joint injuries, such as fractures or ligament tears, increase the risk of osteoarthritis in the affected joint. These injuries can disrupt the normal joint structure and function.

4. Obesity: Excess body weight is a significant risk factor, particularly for osteoarthritis in weight-bearing

joints like the knees and hips. Obesity places added stress on joints and accelerates cartilage degeneration.

5. Joint Overuse: Repetitive movements and activities that strain the joints can lead to osteoarthritis. This is common among individuals with physically demanding jobs or athletes in high-impact sports.

6. Gender: Osteoarthritis is more common in women, especially after menopause. Hormonal changes may play a role in this gender difference.

7. Joint Alignment: Joint deformities or poor alignment can increase the risk of osteoarthritis. Conditions like bowed legs or unequal leg length may contribute to joint stress.

8. Other Medical Conditions: Certain medical conditions, such as rheumatoid arthritis and metabolic disorders, can predispose individuals to osteoarthritis.

Understanding these causes and risk factors allows for better prevention and early intervention strategies. Lifestyle modifications, weight management, and joint protection techniques can help mitigate the risk and reduce the impact of osteoarthritis on individuals' lives.

Osteoarthritis (OA) is a progressive joint disorder, and recognizing its early signs is crucial for timely intervention and management. While OA can affect various joints, such as the knees, hips, hands, and spine, there are common early symptoms to watch for:

1. Joint Pain: Persistent, achy joint pain is often an initial indicator of OA. The pain may be mild initially but can worsen over time, particularly after periods of activity or at the end of the day.

2. Stiffness: Morning joint stiffness that lasts for less than 30 minutes can be an early sign of OA. This stiffness can make it challenging to initiate movement and gradually improve as you get moving throughout the day.

3. Reduced Range of Motion: Early OA may result in a diminished range of motion in the affected joint. This can manifest as difficulty fully bending, straightening, or rotating the joint.

4. Joint Swelling: Swelling around the affected joint is a sign of inflammation, which can occur in response to

OA-related changes. It may be noticeable and tender to the touch.

5. Grating Sensation: In some cases, people with early OA may experience a grating or crunching sensation, known as crepitus, when moving the affected joint. This is due to the roughening of joint surfaces.

Recognizing these early signs of OA can prompt early intervention and lifestyle adjustments, such as weight management, exercise, and joint protection techniques, to help slow the progression of the disease and improve joint function and overall quality of life. If you experience any of these symptoms, it's essential to consult a healthcare professional for a proper evaluation and diagnosis.

Chapter 3

Pathophysiology of Osteoarthritis

Osteoarthritis, often abbreviated as OA, is a complex joint disorder with a well-defined pathophysiology. It involves a cascade of events that ultimately lead to the progressive degeneration of joint structures, particularly the articular cartilage. To understand osteoarthritis's pathophysiology, one must delve into the intricate changes that occur within the affected joints.

Articular Cartilage Breakdown:

The hallmark of osteoarthritis is the gradual erosion of articular cartilage, the smooth, protective tissue covering the ends of bones within a joint. This cartilage acts as a cushion and facilitates frictionless movement. In osteoarthritis, it becomes thinner and less resilient, impairing its ability to perform these essential functions.

.

Cellular Changes:

Within the cartilage, the chondrocytes, specialized cells responsible for maintaining and repairing cartilage, undergo various alterations. These changes can include increased cell death, reduced production of essential extracellular matrix components (such as collagen and proteoglycans), and an imbalance in the processes of cartilage degradation and repair. This results in a net loss of cartilage tissue over time.

Inflammation:

As articular cartilage breaks down, the exposed bone surfaces can become irritated. This irritation leads to a low-grade inflammatory response within the joint. Inflammation contributes to the characteristic joint pain, swelling, and warmth associated with osteoarthritis. Proinflammatory cytokines and enzymes are often elevated in the affected joint.

. Bone RemodelingThe subchondral bone, which lies just beneath the articular cartilage, undergoes changes in response to the cartilage deterioration. It becomes denser and may develop bony outgrowths known as osteophytes or bone spurs. These osteophytes can impede joint movement and cause further discomfort.

Synovial Membrane Changes

:The synovial membrane lines the joint cavity and produces synovial fluid, which lubricates and nourishes the joint. In osteoarthritis, the synovial membrane can become inflamed, a condition known as synovitis. This inflammation leads to increased production of synovial fluid. As a result, the joint may swell and become distended. The excess synovial fluid, rich in inflammatory cytokines, can further perpetuate cartilage damage.

Altered Joint Mechanics:

As the articular cartilage deteriorates, the joint mechanics are disrupted. This can lead to increased friction between joint surfaces, abnormal joint loading, and uneven stress distribution. These mechanical alterations contribute to the overall damage within the joint and further exacerbate the condition.

. Pain and Functional Impairment:

The combined effects of cartilage loss, bone changes, inflammation, and altered joint mechanics result in the hallmark symptoms of osteoarthritis, which include joint pain, stiffness, and reduced mobility. Individuals with osteoarthritis often experience discomfort, especially after periods of inactivity or overuse of the affected joint.

While the precise causes of osteoarthritis are not fully understood, it is believed to be a multifactorial condition. A combination of genetic, mechanical, and environmental factors contributes to its development. Genetics can influence an individual's susceptibility to the disease, while joint injuries, obesity, and repetitive joint use can increase the likelihood of developing osteoarthritis.

Understanding the pathophysiology of osteoarthritis is essential for the development of effective treatment and management strategies. While there is no cure for osteoarthritis, various approaches aim to alleviate pain, improve joint function, and slow disease progression. These may include lifestyle modifications (such as weight management and exercise), pharmacological interventions (pain relievers and anti-inflammatory medications), physical therapy, and, in severe cases, surgical procedures such as joint replacement surgery. In recent years, there has been a growing focus on disease-modifying drugs and regenerative therapies, offering hope for more targeted and advanced treatment options in the future.

Osteoarthritis (OA) is a progressive joint disorder that typically develops through several stages, each marked by increasing severity of symptoms and joint damage. The stages of OA are as follows:

1. Stage 0: Pre-Osteoarthritis - This stage represents a risk factor for OA but does not exhibit any noticeable symptoms or joint damage. It often involves risk factors like family history, joint injuries, or obesity.

2. Stage 1: Minor Cartilage Damage - In this early stage, there may be minor damage to the joint cartilage, but symptoms are usually mild. Joint pain and stiffness might occur after strenuous activity but often resolve with rest.

3. Stage 2: Mild OA - Cartilage loss becomes more apparent, and there may be increased pain, stiffness, and decreased joint flexibility, particularly after activity. X-rays may reveal the presence of osteophytes or bone spurs.

4. Stage 3: Moderate OA - This stage is characterized by more significant cartilage loss, leading to more

noticeable pain and joint stiffness, even during rest. Daily activities may become challenging, and joint deformities may develop.

5. Stage 4: Severe OA - In the final stage, there is substantial cartilage degeneration, joint space narrowing, and pronounced joint deformities. Pain and loss of joint function become severe, affecting daily life and mobility.

It's important to note that not everyone with OA will progress through all these stages, and the rate of progression can vary from person to person. Early diagnosis and appropriate management can help slow the progression of OA and improve the quality of life for individuals affected by this common joint disorder. Consulting a healthcare professional is essential for accurate diagnosis and personalized treatment plans.

Chapter 4

Clinical presentation and symptoms play a pivotal role in diagnosing and managing various medical conditions. When it comes to osteoarthritis, these aspects are key indicators that help healthcare professionals identify and assess the severity of the disease. Osteoarthritis is a degenerative joint disorder primarily affecting the elderly, though it can also occur in younger individuals, especially if they have specific risk factors. Its clinical presentation and symptoms are characteristic and often include the following:

Joint Pain:

Joint pain is the most common and prominent symptom of osteoarthritis. It typically occurs during and after activity, as well as with changes in weather. The pain is usually localized to the affected joint and can vary in intensity. It often presents as a deep, aching discomfort and can be aggravated by weight-bearing activities.

Stiffness:

Joint stiffness is another hallmark of osteoarthritis. Affected individuals often experience morning stiffness, which eases within 30 minutes to an hour. Stiffness can also occur after periods of inactivity, such as sitting for a prolonged duration. It can restrict joint mobility and hinder daily activities.

Reduced Range of Motion:

As osteoarthritis progresses, joint mobility may decrease. Individuals may find it difficult to fully extend or flex the affected joint, which can impact their ability to perform tasks like bending the knee or hip.

Joint Swelling:

Swelling of the joint is a common feature of osteoarthritis. The synovial membrane's inflammation and increased synovial fluid production can result in joint swelling, particularly in more advanced stages of the disease. Swelling often accompanies pain and can make the joint appear larger than normal.

Crepitus:

Crepitus refers to a crackling or grating sensation that occurs within the joint during movement. It is a result of the irregular surfaces of the bones and cartilage rubbing against each other. Crepitus can be both felt and heard by the affected individual.

Joint Deformities:

In advanced osteoarthritis, joint deformities may develop. This can include the formation of osteophytes, or bone spurs, which can alter the joint's appearance and function. In the hands, these bony outgrowths can lead to characteristic finger deformities.

Muscle Weakness:

Due to pain and joint instability, individuals with osteoarthritis may experience muscle weakness around the affected joint. This can lead to functional limitations and difficulty performing everyday activities.

.

Joint Instability:

Joint instability is often reported by those with osteoarthritis, particularly in weight-bearing joints like the knee. This instability can result in a feeling of giving way or buckling, making walking and physical activities more challenging.

Functional Impairment:

Osteoarthritis can significantly impact an individual's ability to perform daily tasks and activities. Difficulty walking, climbing stairs, and getting in and out of chairs are common functional impairments associated with the condition.

Quality of Life Impact:

Beyond the physical symptoms, osteoarthritis can have a substantial impact on an individual's overall quality of life. Chronic pain and reduced mobility can lead to psychological distress, depression, and social isolation.

It's important to note that the clinical presentation and symptoms of osteoarthritis can vary from person to person. The severity and progression of the disease may differ, and some individuals may experience only mild symptoms while others endure more severe discomfort and functional limitations.

Healthcare professionals diagnose osteoarthritis by considering these clinical features and using imaging studies such as X-rays or magnetic resonance imaging (MRI) to confirm joint damage. Early intervention and management are crucial to alleviate symptoms, slow disease progression, and improve the overall well-being of those affected by this common joint disorder. Treatment approaches can include lifestyle modifications, physical therapy, pain management medications, and, in advanced cases, surgical interventions like joint replacement surgery. Understanding the clinical presentation and symptoms is key to providing effective care and support to individuals living with osteoarthritis.

Chapter 5

Diagnosis of Osteoarthritis

Diagnosing osteoarthritis (OA) involves a combination of clinical evaluation, medical history assessment, and diagnostic imaging. It is important to accurately diagnose the condition to implement appropriate management and treatment strategies. The process typically follows a step-by-step approach:

Medical History:

The diagnosis often begins with a comprehensive medical history review. The healthcare provider will ask the patient about their symptoms, the duration of these symptoms, any previous joint injuries, and any relevant family history of joint conditions. Understanding the patient's medical history helps in assessing the risk factors and potential causes of OA.

 Physical ExaminationA thorough physical examination is a crucial step in the diagnostic process. The healthcare provider will assess the affected joint(s) for signs of swelling, tenderness, warmth, and deformities.

They will also evaluate the joint's range of motion, strength, and stability. Joint stiffness and crepitus (crackling or grating sensations during movement) are often noted during the examination.

. Symptom Assessment:

The patient's reported symptoms, such as joint pain, stiffness, and functional limitations, are carefully evaluated. Details about the location, quality, and timing of the pain are important. For OA diagnosis, the pain typically worsens with joint use and improves with rest.

. Imaging Studies:

Diagnostic imaging is a critical component of OA diagnosis. X-rays are commonly used to assess joint damage. X-rays can reveal joint space narrowing, osteophyte formation (bone spurs), and alterations in bone density or shape. These findings are characteristic of OA and help confirm the diagnosis. In some cases, magnetic resonance imaging (MRI) may be used to provide a more detailed view of the joint structures and assess soft tissues like cartilage.

Laboratory Tests:

Unlike other forms of arthritis, such as rheumatoid arthritis, OA does not typically have specific blood markers or laboratory tests to diagnose it. However, blood tests may be ordered to rule out other potential causes of joint symptoms or to assess general health.

. Differential Diagnosis:

To confirm the diagnosis and rule out other possible joint disorders, the healthcare provider may perform a differential diagnosis. This process involves considering other conditions that could mimic OA symptoms, such as rheumatoid arthritis, gout, or septic arthritis. A thorough evaluation is essential to ensure an accurate diagnosis.

Clinical Criteria:

The American College of Rheumatology (ACR) has established clinical criteria for diagnosing hand, hip, and knee osteoarthritis based on clinical and radiographic features. These criteria are used to standardize the diagnosis and research related to OA.

It's worth noting that OA diagnosis primarily relies on clinical evaluation and imaging findings, as there is no definitive blood test or single diagnostic marker for the condition. Accurate diagnosis is essential for tailoring the most appropriate treatment plan.

Osteoarthritis can affect various joints in the body, but it is most commonly diagnosed in weight-bearing joints like the knees and hips, as well as in the hands. The diagnosis can vary depending on the affected joint and the patient's individual circumstances.

The primary goals of diagnosing osteoarthritis are to confirm the condition, assess its severity, and determine the most suitable treatment plan. Once diagnosed, healthcare providers work with patients to develop an individualized management strategy that may include lifestyle modifications, physical therapy, pain management, and, in advanced cases, surgical interventions like joint replacement surgery.

Early diagnosis and intervention are crucial for managing osteoarthritis effectively and improving the quality of life for individuals living with this common joint disorder. It is important to consult with a healthcare provider for a thorough evaluation if you suspect you may have osteoarthritis or are experiencing joint-related symptoms

Laboratory test for osteoarthritis

Diagnosing osteoarthritis (OA) typically involves a combination of clinical assessment, medical history, and imaging studies. Laboratory tests are less commonly used for OA diagnosis but may be helpful in ruling out other conditions that could be causing joint symptoms. Here are some laboratory tests that might be considered:

1. **Blood Tests**: Blood tests are often used to rule out other types of arthritis, such as rheumatoid arthritis. Elevated levels of certain markers, like rheumatoid factor and anti-cyclic citrullinated peptide (anti-CCP) antibodies, are associated with other forms of arthritis but are not typically found in OA.

2. **Joint Fluid Analysis**: In some cases, joint aspiration or synovial fluid analysis may be performed to rule out infections or crystal-induced arthropathies (e.g., gout). OA joint fluid usually appears clear and does not show the presence of uric acid crystals or signs of infection.

3. **Inflammatory Markers**: Blood tests may include markers like C-reactive protein (CRP) and erythrocyte sedimentation rate (ESR) to assess the presence of inflammation. Elevated levels may indicate inflammatory arthritis rather than OA.

While laboratory tests can be valuable for ruling out other conditions that mimic OA, the primary diagnostic methods for OA typically involve physical examination and imaging techniques, such as X-rays and MRI scans, to assess joint structure and confirm the diagnosis. A healthcare professional will use a combination of these diagnostic tools to determine whether OA is the cause of a patient's joint pain and stiffness

Chapter 6

Management and Treatment

Management and treatment of osteoarthritis (OA) aim to alleviate pain, improve joint function, and enhance the overall quality of life for individuals affected by this common joint disorder. The approach to managing OA is typically multifaceted and tailored to the individual's specific needs and the severity of their condition. Here is an overview of the various management and treatment options for osteoarthritis:

. Lifestyle Modifications:

Weight Management:

Maintaining a healthy weight is crucial for OA management, especially in weight-bearing joints like the knees and hips. Excess weight places additional stress on joints, exacerbating symptoms. Weight loss, achieved through a combination of dietary changes and regular exercise, can significantly reduce pain and improve function.

Exercise:

Regular physical activity is essential for OA management. Exercise helps to strengthen the muscles around the affected joints, improve joint flexibility, and maintain overall joint health. Low-impact activities like swimming, walking, and cycling are generally recommended. Physical therapy can also be beneficial to learn specific exercises and techniques for joint protection.

Assistive Devices:

Assistive devices such as canes, braces, and orthotic shoe inserts can help reduce joint stress and improve stability, making it easier for individuals to perform daily activities.

Joint Protection:

Learning proper techniques for joint protection during activities of daily living can help reduce joint strain. This may involve ergonomic adjustments to workspaces or using adaptive tools to ease the load on joints.

Medications

-Pain Relievers: Over-the-counter pain relievers such as acetaminophen can help manage mild to moderate OA pain. Nonsteroidal anti-inflammatory drugs (NSAIDs) may be prescribed for more severe pain and inflammation. However, long-term use of NSAIDs can have side effects and should be monitored closely by a healthcare provider.

Topical Analgesics:

Topical creams and gels that contain NSAIDs or capsaicin can provide localized pain relief without the potential systemic side effects of oral medications.

Intra-Articular Injections:

Corticosteroid injections directly into the affected joint can provide temporary pain relief and reduce inflammation. Hyaluronic acid injections, also known as viscosupplementation, can help lubricate the joint and alleviate pain.

Disease-Modifying Osteoarthritis Drugs (DMOADs):

These are a newer class of medications designed to slow the progression of OA. One example is hyaluronic acid derivatives that may help improve joint health.

Surgical Interventions:

Arthroscopy:

In some cases, arthroscopic surgery may be performed to clean out or repair damaged joint tissues. However, the effectiveness of arthroscopy for OA is debated, and it is not typically recommended for advanced cases.

Joint Replacement Surgery:

Joint replacement surgery, such as hip or knee replacement, is considered when OA is severe and significantly impairs an individual's quality of life. During the procedure, the damaged joint is replaced with an artificial joint (prosthesis), which can restore joint function and alleviate pain.

. Complementary and Alternative Therapies:

Acupuncture: Some individuals with OA find relief from acupuncture, a practice that involves the insertion of thin needles into specific points on the body.

Dietary Supplements: Glucosamine and chondroitin sulfate are commonly used dietary supplements to promote joint health. While evidence on their effectiveness is mixed, some people report symptom improvement.

Herbal Remedies:Herbal supplements like turmeric and Boswellia have anti-inflammatory properties and may help reduce OA symptoms. However, their effectiveness varies, and it's important to consult with a healthcare provider before using herbal remedies.

Self-Management Strategies:

Education: Understanding the condition and how to manage it is essential. Education can empower individuals to make informed decisions about their care.

Self-Care: Heat and cold therapy, as well as using joint supports like braces, can provide relief. Additionally, self-massage and maintaining a healthy sleep routine can be beneficial.

Monitoring:Regularly monitoring symptoms and seeking prompt medical attention for changes or complications is important.

Research and Emerging Therapies:

Ongoing research is exploring new treatments for osteoarthritis, including the development of disease-modifying drugs, regenerative therapies (such as stem cell treatments), and innovative surgical techniques. These therapies hold promise for the future of OA management.

It's essential to note that there is no one-size-fits-all approach to treating osteoarthritis.

Management and treatment plans should be individualized, taking into account factors like the affected joints, disease severity, age, and overall health. Furthermore, managing osteoarthritis often involves a combination of these strategies, and treatment plans may evolve over time as the condition progresses.

A multidisciplinary approach, involving healthcare providers, physical therapists, occupational therapists, and, in some cases, pain management specialists or rheumatologists, is often the most effective way to address the complexities of osteoarthritis.

Moreover, lifestyle modifications, such as weight management and exercise, are foundational components of osteoarthritis management, as they can significantly impact symptom relief and the overall progression of the disease. While there is no cure for osteoarthritis, effective management and treatment can help individuals lead fulfilling lives and maintain their independence despite the challenges posed by this common joint disorder.

-

Medications play a crucial role in the management of osteoarthritis by providing pain relief, reducing inflammation, and improving joint function. Pain relievers like acetaminophen and nonsteroidal anti-inflammatory drugs (NSAIDs) help individuals manage discomfort, enhancing their quality of life. In cases of severe pain and inflammation, intra-articular injections or disease-modifying osteoarthritis drugs (DMOADs) may be recommended to provide targeted relief or slow disease progression. While medications do not cure osteoarthritis, they are vital for symptom control and can enable individuals to engage in physical therapy and maintain an active lifestyle, ultimately improving their overall well-being.

Pain Relief Medications

Pain relief medications are a fundamental aspect of osteoarthritis (OA) management, as they provide much-needed relief from the chronic discomfort associated with the condition. These medications aim to alleviate pain, reduce inflammation, and improve an individual's overall quality of life. Here are the primary pain relief medications commonly used for OA:

1. Acetaminophen (Tylenol):

Acetaminophen is often the first-line pain reliever recommended for mild to moderate OA. It works by reducing pain perception in the brain and has anti-inflammatory properties. It's considered a safer option for those who cannot tolerate NSAIDs due to gastrointestinal issues. However, it should be used cautiously and within recommended dosage limits, as excessive intake can harm the liver.

2. Nonsteroidal Anti-Inflammatory Drugs (NSAIDs):

NSAIDs are commonly used for moderate to severe OA pain and inflammation. They work by reducing inflammation and blocking pain signals. Over-the-counter options like ibuprofen (Advil) and naproxen (Aleve) are available, as well as prescription-strength NSAIDs. Long-term use may carry risks, including gastrointestinal problems and cardiovascular side effects, so healthcare providers closely monitor their use.

3. Cyclooxygenase-2 (COX-2) Inhibitors:

COX-2 inhibitors are a subclass of NSAIDs that specifically target the cyclooxygenase-2 enzyme, which is responsible for inflammation and pain. Medications like celecoxib (Celebrex) offer pain relief with potentially fewer gastrointestinal side effects, making them suitable for some individuals.

4. Topical Analgesics: Topical creams, gels, or patches containing NSAIDs (e.g., diclofenac) or capsaicin can be applied directly to the skin over the affected joint. These topical agents offer localized pain relief without the systemic side effects associated with oral medications.

5. Intra-Articular Injections:

For individuals with OA in specific joints, such as the knee, corticosteroid injections into the joint can provide temporary pain relief and reduce inflammation. Hyaluronic acid injections, known as viscosupplementation, can help lubricate the joint and alleviate pain, though their effectiveness is a subject of debate.

It's essential to consult with a healthcare provider to determine the most suitable pain relief medication and to closely monitor its use. They can assess the severity of symptoms, the individual's overall health, and any potential contraindications to make informed treatment decisions.

While pain relief medications can significantly improve the quality of life for individuals with OA, they do not address the underlying disease process. Therefore, a comprehensive management plan often involves additional strategies, such as lifestyle modifications, physical therapy, assistive devices, and in some cases, surgical interventions.

Medications are an essential tool in the multifaceted approach to osteoarthritis management. They help individuals manage pain, regain mobility, and lead active lives despite the challenges posed by this common joint disorder.

Disease-Modifying Osteoarthritis

Disease-Modifying Osteoarthritis Drugs (DMOADs) are a class of medications designed to slow the progression of osteoarthritis (OA) by targeting the underlying disease processes. Unlike pain relief medications, which primarily manage symptoms, DMOADs aim to modify the course of the disease. Examples include hyaluronic acid derivatives that may help improve joint health by enhancing the quality of synovial fluid and promoting cartilage preservation. While their effectiveness is still a subject of research and debate, DMOADs hold promise as a potential means to delay the joint damage seen in OA and improve long-term outcomes for individuals affected by this chronic joint condition.

Examples of Disease-Modifying Osteoarthritis and uses

Disease-Modifying Osteoarthritis Drugs (DMOADs) are a relatively new class of medications aimed at slowing the progression of osteoarthritis (OA) by targeting the underlying mechanisms of the disease. While research is ongoing, several promising DMOADs and their potential uses have emerged:

1. Hyaluronic Acid Derivatives (Viscosupplementation): Hyaluronic acid is a natural component of synovial fluid that lubricates and cushions the joints. In OA, the quality and quantity of hyaluronic acid are often reduced. Viscosupplementation involves injecting hyaluronic acid derivatives directly into the affected joint. These injections aim to restore the joint's lubricating properties, reduce pain, and potentially slow down cartilage degeneration. Viscosupplementation is most commonly used for knee OA, and its use can improve joint function and provide pain relief.

2. Diacerein: Diacerein is an oral medication that has shown potential as a DMOAD. It may help inhibit the enzymes responsible for breaking down cartilage in OA joints. Diacerein has been studied in knee and hip OA, and while it may slow disease progression, its effects are generally modest. It is available in some regions, but its use is subject to ongoing research and regulatory considerations.

3.*Strontium Ranelate: Strontium ranelate is a medication used for the treatment of osteoporosis that has shown potential for OA. It is believed to stimulate cartilage growth while inhibiting bone resorption. Studies have suggested that strontium ranelate can slow cartilage loss and reduce pain in knee OA. However, its use for OA is not widely approved, and further research is needed.

4. Platelet-Rich Plasma (PRP):PRP is an autologous blood product that contains a concentrated amount of platelets, growth factors, and cytokines. It is prepared by drawing the patient's blood, processing it to extract the platelet-rich portion, and then injecting it into the OA-affected joint. PRP may promote cartilage regeneration and reduce inflammation, potentially serving as a DMOAD. Research on PRP's effectiveness in OA management, particularly for knee OA, is ongoing.

5. Stem Cell Therapies: Stem cell-based therapies are an exciting area of research in the field of DMOADs. Autologous mesenchymal stem cells (MSCs) have shown promise in preclinical and early clinical studies for OA. MSCs have the potential to differentiate into various joint tissues and promote healing. These therapies are still in the experimental stage and require further research and regulatory approvals.

It's important to note that while these DMOADs hold promise, the effectiveness of these treatments may vary between individuals and specific joints. DMOADs are often considered for individuals with moderate to severe OA and may be used in combination with other conservative treatments.

Patients should consult with their healthcare provider to discuss the potential benefits, risks, and appropriate DMOAD options based on their specific OA symptoms and needs. Additionally, ongoing research is vital to refine the understanding and use of DMOADs in osteoarthritis management, with the ultimate goal of improving the lives of those affected by this common joint disorder

Chapter 7

Non-Pharmacological Approaches

Non-Pharmacological Approaches for Osteoarthritis Management

Osteoarthritis (OA) is a common degenerative joint disease that affects millions of people worldwide. It primarily targets the articular cartilage, causing pain, stiffness, and reduced joint function. While pharmaceutical interventions like painkillers and anti-inflammatory drugs can help manage the symptoms, they often come with side effects and do not address the root cause of OA. Non-pharmacological approaches are increasingly recognized as vital components of OA management, focusing on lifestyle modifications, exercise, physical therapies, and other holistic techniques. In this article, we will explore the importance and effectiveness of non-pharmacological approaches for managing osteoarthritis.

1. Exercise and Physical Activity

Regular physical activity plays a crucial role in managing osteoarthritis. It helps maintain joint mobility and muscle strength, which can alleviate pain and improve overall joint function. Low-impact exercises such as swimming, walking, and cycling are often recommended for individuals with OA, as they reduce joint stress while promoting cardiovascular fitness. Physical therapists can design tailored exercise programs that address specific joint limitations and gradually build strength.

2. Weight Management:

Excess body weight is a significant risk factor for OA, especially in weight-bearing joints like the knees and hips. Weight management is a non-pharmacological approach that involves maintaining a healthy body mass to reduce the strain on affected joints. A combination of dietary modifications and regular exercise can help individuals with OA achieve and maintain a healthy weight, thus reducing the progression of the disease and its associated symptoms.

3. Dietary Modifications:

While there is no specific diet to cure osteoarthritis, certain dietary choices can help manage symptoms.

Omega-3 fatty acids, found in fish and flaxseed, have anti-inflammatory properties and may provide some relief. Antioxidant-rich foods, such as fruits and vegetables, can help reduce oxidative stress and support joint health. Additionally, limiting processed foods and foods high in sugar and trans fats may help reduce inflammation.

4. Physical Therapy:

Physical therapy is a key non-pharmacological approach for managing osteoarthritis. It involves a range of techniques, including manual therapy, joint mobilization, and therapeutic exercises, to improve joint function and reduce pain. Physical therapists work closely with patients to develop personalized treatment plans that address their specific needs and limitations.

5. Assistive Devices:

Assistive devices, such as braces, splints, and orthotic inserts, can provide support and stability to affected joints. They are particularly helpful for individuals with OA in weight-bearing joints. By redistributing pressure and providing added support, these devices can reduce pain and improve mobility.

6. Heat and Cold Therapy:

Heat and cold therapy are simple yet effective methods for managing OA symptoms. Heat therapy can relax muscles and increase blood flow to the affected area, while cold therapy can reduce inflammation and numb pain. Patients can alternate between these treatments to find the most effective relief for their specific symptoms.

7. Acupuncture:

Acupuncture is an alternative therapy that involves inserting thin needles into specific points on the body. Some studies suggest that acupuncture may help reduce OA-related pain and improve joint function. While the exact mechanisms behind its effectiveness are not fully understood, many individuals with OA report relief after acupuncture sessions.

8. Mind-Body Techniques:

Mind-body techniques such as meditation, mindfulness, and relaxation exercises can help individuals with OA manage the emotional and psychological aspects of chronic pain. These techniques can reduce stress and anxiety, which are known to exacerbate OA symptoms. By promoting a sense of calm and relaxation, mind-body practices can complement other non-pharmacological approaches.

9. Education and Self-Management:

Patient education is a critical component of osteoarthritis management. By understanding their condition and learning how to manage it effectively, individuals can take an active role in their care. Self-management strategies may include joint protection techniques, pain management strategies, and lifestyle modifications.

10.Occupational Therapy:

Occupational therapists can assist individuals with OA in adapting their daily activities to minimize joint stress and maximize function. They can recommend assistive devices, ergonomic modifications, and techniques to conserve energy and reduce the impact of OA on daily life.

In conclusion, non-pharmacological approaches are essential components of osteoarthritis management. These approaches encompass a wide range of techniques, from exercise and weight management to physical therapy, dietary modifications, and alternative therapies. When used in combination, these approaches can help individuals with OA effectively manage their symptoms, improve joint function, and enhance their overall quality of life. It's important to note that the effectiveness of these approaches may vary from person to person, and consultation with healthcare professionals is crucial for developing personalized treatment plans. By incorporating non-pharmacological strategies into their daily routines, individuals with osteoarthritis can better control the impact of this chronic condition on their lives.i

Chapter 8

Pharmacological Management

Osteoarthritis (OA) is a common degenerative joint disease that affects millions of people worldwide. It is characterized by the progressive deterioration of joint cartilage, leading to pain, stiffness, and reduced mobility. While non-pharmacological interventions, such as physical therapy and lifestyle modifications, play a crucial role in managing OA, pharmacological approaches are often necessary to alleviate symptoms and improve patients' quality of life. This article explores the various pharmacological options available for the management of osteoarthritis.

1. Nonsteroidal Anti-Inflammatory Drugs (NSAIDs):

NSAIDs are commonly used for the management of OA due to their ability to relieve pain and reduce inflammation. These medications work by inhibiting enzymes responsible for producing prostaglandins, which are chemicals that promote pain and inflammation. Both over-the-counter (OTC) and prescription NSAIDs are available, and they can be taken orally or applied topically as creams or gels.

Popular NSAIDs include ibuprofen, naproxen, and diclofenac.

While NSAIDs can provide effective pain relief, they are not without side effects. Gastrointestinal issues, such as stomach ulcers and bleeding, are common concerns with long-term NSAID use. Additionally, NSAIDs can increase the risk of cardiovascular events, such as heart attacks and strokes. Therefore, they should be used cautiously, and patients with a history of gastrointestinal or cardiovascular problems should consult with their healthcare providers before using NSAIDs.

2. Acetaminophen:

Acetaminophen, commonly known as paracetamol, is another over-the-counter pain reliever often used to manage osteoarthritis. Unlike NSAIDs, acetaminophen does not have anti-inflammatory properties. Instead, it works by reducing pain perception in the brain. Acetaminophen is generally well-tolerated and is a suitable option for individuals who cannot tolerate NSAIDs due to gastrointestinal or cardiovascular concerns.

However, it's essential to be cautious when using acetaminophen, as high doses can lead to liver damage. Patients should follow the recommended dosage and avoid combining acetaminophen with alcohol, as it can increase the risk of liver problems.

3. Intra-Articular Corticosteroid Injections:

In cases where osteoarthritis symptoms are localized to a specific joint, intra-articular corticosteroid injections may be considered. This treatment involves injecting a corticosteroid directly into the affected joint. Corticosteroids have potent anti-inflammatory properties and can provide rapid relief from pain and inflammation.

Intra-articular corticosteroid injections are a suitable option for patients with moderate to severe osteoarthritis who have not responded well to oral medications. However, they are typically used as a short-term solution, as repeated injections may lead to joint damage. Potential side effects of corticosteroid injections include temporary pain and swelling at the injection site, as well as rare complications like joint infection.

4. Disease-Modifying Osteoarthritis Drugs (DMOADs):

Unlike some other forms of arthritis, OA has not traditionally been associated with disease-modifying drugs, but there are ongoing efforts to develop pharmaceutical treatments that can slow down the progression of the disease. Some potential DMOADs under investigation include sprifermin, which stimulates cartilage growth, and anti-nerve growth factor antibodies, which may reduce pain.

5. Hyaluronic Acid Injections:

Hyaluronic acid is a natural component of joint fluid that helps lubricate and cushion the joint. In osteoarthritis, the quality and quantity of hyaluronic acid in the joint may be reduced. Hyaluronic acid injections, also known as viscosupplementation, involve injecting a gel-like substance into the joint to restore its lubricating properties and reduce pain.

Hyaluronic acid injections are most effective for individuals with knee osteoarthritis, and the treatment typically involves a series of injections over several weeks. While they are generally well-tolerated, some patients may experience temporary pain and swelling at the injection site.

6. Opioids:

Opioid medications are powerful pain relievers that may be prescribed for severe osteoarthritis pain when other treatments have not provided adequate relief. However, due to the risk of dependence and addiction associated with opioids, their use in osteoarthritis is controversial. Healthcare providers typically reserve opioid prescriptions for cases where other options have been exhausted and closely monitor patients to minimize the potential for misuse.

7. Topical Analgesics:

Topical analgesics, such as creams, gels, and patches, can provide localized pain relief for osteoarthritis. These products often contain ingredients like capsaicin, menthol, or salicylates and work by numbing the skin and underlying tissues. They are particularly useful for people with OA in the hands, knees, or other superficial joints.

In conclusion, pharmacological management plays a significant role in alleviating the pain and discomfort associated with osteoarthritis. However, it is crucial for healthcare providers to tailor treatment plans to individual patients, taking into consideration their overall health, comorbid conditions, and potential side effects.

Additionally, patients should be educated about the benefits and risks of various medications and actively participate in shared decision-making with their healthcare team to ensure the most appropriate and effective management of their osteoarthritis symptoms.

Chapter 9

Surgical Interventions

Osteoarthritis (OA) is a debilitating joint disease that affects millions of individuals worldwide. While non-surgical methods such as pharmacological management, physical therapy, and lifestyle modifications play a significant role in treating OA, there are cases where surgical interventions become necessary. This article explores the various surgical procedures and interventions used in the management of osteoarthritis.

Surgery for osteoarthritis is typically considered when conservative treatments have failed to provide adequate relief, and the pain and loss of joint function significantly impact the patient's quality of life. The choice of surgical intervention depends on several factors, including the affected joint, the extent of cartilage damage, the patient's overall health, and their preferences. Below are some of the common surgical interventions for osteoarthritis:

1. Arthroscopy:

Arthroscopy is a minimally invasive surgical procedure used for both the diagnosis and treatment of osteoarthritis, primarily in the knee joint. During an arthroscopic procedure, the surgeon makes small incisions and inserts a thin, flexible tube with a camera (arthroscope) into the joint. This allows them to visualize the joint's interior and assess the extent of cartilage damage. In some cases, minor surgical corrections, such as smoothing out rough cartilage or removing loose fragments, can be performed during the same procedure.

While arthroscopy can provide short-term relief for some patients, it is not a long-term solution for osteoarthritis. The benefits of arthroscopy may vary from person to person, and it is typically considered when conservative treatments have not been effective or when there are mechanical issues within the joint.

2. Osteotomy:

An osteotomy is a surgical procedure used to correct joint alignment by reshaping the bones around the affected joint. This procedure is commonly performed on the knee and hip joints and is most often recommended for younger patients with early-stage osteoarthritis. By changing the alignment of the joint, osteotomy can help redistribute the load on the affected area, relieving pain and slowing down the progression of osteoarthritis.

Knee osteotomy, for example, involves removing a wedge of bone from either the femur (thigh bone) or tibia (shin bone) to shift the weight-bearing forces away from the damaged part of the knee joint. Hip osteotomy, on the other hand, focuses on repositioning the hip socket to improve stability and reduce cartilage wear.

While osteotomies can be effective in delaying the need for joint replacement, they are not suitable for all patients, and the recovery process can be lengthy. Moreover, osteotomies do not guarantee a complete cure and may need to be followed by other surgical interventions as OA progresses.

3. Joint Resurfacing:

Joint resurfacing, also known as surface replacement or cartilage repair surgery, is a procedure that focuses on preserving the damaged joint's natural structure and function. This technique is most commonly used for hip and shoulder joints, and it involves removing and replacing the worn-out cartilage and damaged bone while preserving as much healthy bone as possible. Resurfacing aims to provide pain relief and restore joint mobility.

Hip resurfacing, for instance, involves capping the femoral head with a metal prosthesis while preserving more of the patient's natural bone compared to a traditional total hip replacement. Shoulder resurfacing is similar in concept, as it involves replacing the worn-out cartilage with a metal implant that replicates the natural joint's shape.

Joint resurfacing is generally recommended for patients with early-stage osteoarthritis, good bone quality, and healthy surrounding tissues. It may offer advantages like improved range of motion and reduced risk of dislocation compared to traditional joint replacement procedures. However, not all patients are candidates for joint resurfacing, and the long-term durability of the implants is a subject of ongoing research.

4. Total Joint Replacement (Arthroplasty):
Total joint replacement, also known as arthroplasty, is one of the most common and effective surgical interventions for advanced osteoarthritis. This procedure involves removing the damaged joint components and replacing them with artificial implants made of metal, plastic, or ceramic materials. Total joint replacement can be performed on various joints, including the hip, knee, shoulder, and elbow.

The goal of total joint replacement is to relieve pain, restore joint function, and improve the patient's quality of life. The procedure typically results in significant pain relief and improved mobility, allowing patients to return to their daily activities and enjoy a better quality of life.

Hip replacement surgery, for example, involves replacing the hip joint's femoral head and the acetabulum (hip socket) with artificial components. Knee replacement replaces the damaged surfaces of the femur, tibia, and patella. Shoulder replacement can involve replacing the humeral head or the glenoid (shoulder socket).

The success rate of total joint replacement is generally high, and patients often experience significant improvements in pain relief and function. However, it is a major surgery with potential risks and complications, including infection, blood clots, and implant wear. Rehabilitation and physical therapy are essential components of the recovery process to ensure the best outcomes.

5. Partial Joint Replacement (Hemi-arthroplasty):

Partial joint replacement, or hemi-arthroplasty, involves replacing only one part of a joint, typically the damaged or degenerated component. This procedure is often used in cases where only one side of the joint is affected by osteoarthritis. For example, hemi-arthroplasty can be performed on the hip or shoulder, replacing the femoral head or humeral head while preserving the natural socket.

Partial joint replacement is generally recommended when the joint's cartilage damage is localized, and the patient's overall health and joint function can benefit from preserving as much natural bone as possible. This procedure can provide significant pain relief and improved function while maintaining the patient's joint stability.

6. Revision Surgery:

In some cases, patients may require revision surgery due to complications, implant wear, or other issues arising after a joint replacement procedure. Revision surgery involves removing and replacing the existing artificial implants. This type of surgery is typically more complex and challenging than the initial joint replacement and may require specialized components and techniques.

Revision surgery is essential to address issues such as implant loosening, infection, implant wear, and instability. The goal of revision surgery is to restore the patient's pain relief, joint function, and overall satisfaction. The specific approach and components used in revision surgery depend on the individual circumstances and challenges encountered.

In conclusion, surgical interventions play a crucial role in the management of osteoarthritis, particularly in cases where non-surgical treatments have not provided sufficient relief. The choice of surgical procedure depends on the affected joint, the extent of cartilage damage, the patient's overall health, and their individual goals and preferences. While surgical interventions can significantly improve the quality of life for individuals with osteoarthritis, they should always be carefully considered and discussed with a healthcare provider to ensure the most appropriate and effective treatment plan. Furthermore, ongoing advancements in surgical techniques and implant materials continue to enhance the outcomes and longevity of joint surgeries, offering hope for improved management of osteoarthritis in the future.

Living and coping with osteoarthritis

Living and coping with osteoarthritis (OA) can be challenging, but with proper management and lifestyle adjustments, individuals can lead fulfilling lives while minimizing the impact of this chronic joint condition.

1. **Pain Management**: Pain is a common and often debilitating symptom of OA. Over-the-counter pain relievers or prescribed medications can help manage pain. Non-steroidal anti-inflammatory drugs (NSAIDs) and acetaminophen are commonly used, but long-term use should be monitored by a healthcare provider.

2. **Physical Activity**: Regular, low-impact exercise is crucial for maintaining joint function and reducing pain. Activities like swimming, walking, and gentle stretching can help strengthen the muscles around affected joints, improve flexibility, and support overall joint health.

3. **Weight Management**: Maintaining a healthy weight is essential because excess weight puts additional stress on weight-bearing joints like the knees and hips. Losing weight, if necessary, can significantly alleviate symptoms.

4. **Assistive Devices**: Devices like canes, braces, or shoe inserts can provide support and reduce joint strain.

Mobility aids like walkers or wheelchairs may be beneficial in severe cases.

5. **Physical Therapy**: Working with a physical therapist can provide personalized exercise programs, manual therapy, and guidance on proper body mechanics to manage OA effectively.

6. **Diet and Nutrition**: A balanced diet rich in anti-inflammatory foods can help manage inflammation and support joint health. Omega-3 fatty acids, found in fatty fish and flaxseed, may have anti-inflammatory properties.

7. **Mind-Body Techniques**: Relaxation techniques such as yoga, meditation, and deep breathing exercises can help manage stress and improve overall well-being, potentially reducing the perception of pain.

Coping with OA often involves a multi-faceted approach, and each person's experience is unique. Engaging with healthcare professionals, such as rheumatologists and physical therapists, is essential for developing a personalized management plan. With the right strategies and support, individuals can maintain an active and fulfilling lifestyle while effectively managing the challenges of osteoarthritis.

Chapter 10

Complications and Comorbidities

Osteoarthritis (OA) is a degenerative joint disease that primarily affects the articular cartilage of joints, leading to pain, stiffness, and reduced mobility. While the disease primarily targets the joints, it can have far-reaching consequences for a patient's overall health. In this article, we will explore the complications and comorbidities associated with osteoarthritis.

Complications of Osteoarthritis

1. Chronic Pain: The hallmark symptom of osteoarthritis is chronic joint pain. Over time, the persistent pain can lead to physical and psychological complications. It can limit a person's ability to perform daily activities, decrease their quality of life, and even result in depression and anxiety. The ongoing pain can disrupt sleep, leading to sleep disturbances and further impacting one's overall well-being.

2. Loss of Mobility: Osteoarthritis often leads to joint stiffness and a reduced range of motion. As the disease progresses, patients may find it increasingly challenging to perform simple tasks, such as walking, climbing

stairs, or bending. Loss of mobility can negatively impact independence and reduce one's overall quality of life.

3. Muscle Weakness: The pain and reduced mobility associated with osteoarthritis can result in muscle weakness, as patients may avoid using the affected joint to minimize discomfort. Muscle atrophy and weakness can further exacerbate joint problems, creating a vicious cycle of pain and physical decline.

4. Joint Deformities: In advanced cases of osteoarthritis, joint deformities can develop. Deformities can affect the alignment and stability of the joint, causing further pain and limiting function. For example, in knee osteoarthritis, a common deformity is the "bowleg" or "knock-knee" appearance.

5. Gait Abnormalities: Osteoarthritis can alter a person's gait, leading to an abnormal walking pattern. This can put extra stress on other joints and increase the risk of falls, further complicating the patient's condition.

6. Secondary Infections: Joint deformities, skin breakdown, and open wounds in advanced osteoarthritis can increase the risk of secondary infections, including cellulitis and septic arthritis. These infections can lead to severe complications and require immediate medical attention.

7. Osteophytes: Osteoarthritis can lead to the formation of bone spurs or osteophytes. These bony outgrowths can impinge on adjacent structures, causing pain and restricted joint movement.

Comorbidities Associated with Osteoarthritis:

1. Cardiovascular Diseases: There is a well-established association between osteoarthritis and cardiovascular diseases such as hypertension, heart disease, and stroke. Chronic inflammation, a common feature of osteoarthritis, may contribute to the development and progression of cardiovascular conditions.

2. Obesity: Osteoarthritis is closely linked to obesity. Excess body weight puts added stress on weight-bearing joints, especially the knees and hips. Obesity increases the risk of developing osteoarthritis and exacerbates the severity of the disease in those already affected.

3. Metabolic Syndrome Osteoarthritis is also linked to metabolic syndrome, a cluster of conditions that include high blood pressure, high blood sugar, excess abdominal fat, and abnormal cholesterol levels.

Metabolic syndrome is a risk factor for cardiovascular disease and type 2 diabetes.

4. Diabetes: While the exact relationship is complex, there is a bidirectional connection between diabetes and osteoarthritis. Individuals with diabetes are at an increased risk of developing osteoarthritis, and osteoarthritis may contribute to the development of insulin resistance and impaired glucose metabolism.

5. Depression and Anxiety: Chronic pain, disability, and limitations in daily activities can lead to mental health issues. Depression and anxiety are common comorbidities in osteoarthritis, affecting both the patient's overall quality of life and their ability to adhere to treatment plans.

6. Osteoporosis: Osteoarthritis and osteoporosis share risk factors, such as age and hormonal changes. Osteoporosis, characterized by a decrease in bone density, can coexist with osteoarthritis and increase the risk of fractures, further complicating the clinical picture.

7.Fractures:Individuals with osteoarthritis may be at an increased risk of fractures, particularly hip fractures. Reduced joint stability and muscle weakness can contribute to falls and fractures in older adults.

8. Cancer :Some studies suggest a link between osteoarthritis and certain types of cancer, such as colon and breast cancer. The mechanisms underlying this association are not fully understood and require further investigation.

9. Chronic Kidney Disease: There is evidence to suggest that individuals with osteoarthritis may be at a higher risk of developing chronic kidney disease, although the exact relationship is complex and not fully elucidated.

10. Sleep Disturbances: Pain and discomfort associated with osteoarthritis can lead to sleep disturbances, exacerbating fatigue and impairing overall well-being.

Managing Complications and Comorbidities:

Effective management of osteoarthritis requires a comprehensive approach that considers not only the joint disease but also its associated complications and comorbidities. Some key strategies for managing complications and comorbidities include:

Pain Management: Effective pain management is critical. This may involve a combination of pharmacological interventions, physical therapy, and lifestyle modifications.

Exercise and Physical Therapy: Strengthening the muscles around affected joints can help improve mobility, reduce pain, and prevent further complications.

Weight Management: Maintaining a healthy weight is essential, particularly for individuals with obesity. Weight loss can reduce stress on weight-bearing joints and improve overall health.

 Mental Health Support: Addressing depression and anxiety through counseling, support groups, or medication can improve the patient's mental well-being.

Regular Monitoring: Patients with osteoarthritis and comorbidities should receive regular medical check-ups to monitor their overall health and address any emerging issues promptly.
Medication Management: For individuals with comorbid conditions like diabetes or hypertension, proper medication management is essential. Coordination between healthcare providers is vital to optimize treatment.

In conclusion, osteoarthritis is not an isolated joint condition but can lead to various complications and comorbidities that affect an individual's overall health and well-being. It is crucial to take a holistic approach to manage these associated issues in conjunction with addressing the primary joint disease. Multidisciplinary care and a patient-centered approach are essential to provide comprehensive and effective management for individuals living with osteoarthritis and its related complications and comorbidities.

Chapter 11

Prevention and Lifestyle Guidelines

Preventing osteoarthritis and managing its symptoms often begins with lifestyle choices. Regular exercise, maintaining a healthy weight, and protecting your joints can help prevent the development or progression of the disease. Incorporating low-impact activities, such as swimming or cycling, can strengthen muscles and improve joint flexibility. A balanced diet rich in nutrients supports joint health, while weight management reduces the stress on weight-bearing joints. Additionally, practicing proper ergonomics, protecting joints during physical activities, and avoiding overuse can reduce the risk of osteoarthritis. Lifestyle changes that promote joint health are key to preventing and managing this common joint condition.

Preventing Osteoarthritis

Osteoarthritis is a degenerative joint disease that can lead to chronic pain, reduced mobility, and a significant decline in the quality of life. While some risk factors, such as age and genetics, cannot be controlled, there are steps individuals can take to reduce their risk of developing osteoarthritis and slow its progression. Here are essential strategies for preventing osteoarthritis:

1. Maintain a Healthy Weight: Excess weight places additional stress on weight-bearing joints, such as the knees and hips. Losing weight or maintaining a healthy weight can significantly reduce the risk of osteoarthritis development and alleviate symptoms in individuals already affected.

2. Regular Exercise: Engaging in regular, low-impact exercises is crucial for maintaining joint health. Activities like swimming, cycling, and walking help strengthen the muscles around joints, improve flexibility, and provide support to the joint structures.

3. Protect Your Joints: Be mindful of joint protection techniques, such as using assistive devices when needed, maintaining proper posture, and avoiding excessive or repetitive stress on joints during physical activities.

4. Adequate Nutrition: A balanced diet rich in vitamins and minerals, including calcium and vitamin D, supports strong bones and joints. Omega-3 fatty acids, found in foods like fish, have anti-inflammatory properties that can help reduce joint inflammation.

5. Avoid Joint Injuries: Preventing joint injuries is essential. This involves practicing safe techniques during sports and physical activities, wearing appropriate protective gear, and being cautious to prevent accidents that may damage joints.

6. Healthy Lifestyle Choices: Avoid smoking, which has been linked to an increased risk of developing osteoarthritis. Excessive alcohol consumption can also contribute to joint damage, so moderation is key.

7. Regular Health Check-ups: Early detection of joint issues can help in the timely management of osteoarthritis. Regular check-ups with a healthcare provider can identify risk factors and monitor joint health.

Incorporating these preventive measures into your lifestyle can significantly reduce the risk of osteoarthritis development and provide a foundation for better joint health in the long term. Remember that it's essential to consult with a healthcare professional for personalized guidance and recommendations based on your specific circumstances and risk factors

Coping with Osteoarthritis

Osteoarthritis can be a challenging and sometimes debilitating condition, but there are several strategies that individuals can employ to effectively cope with the disease and maintain a good quality of life.

1. Pain Management: Managing pain is a central aspect of coping with osteoarthritis. Over-the-counter or prescription pain relievers, physical therapy, and lifestyle modifications can help alleviate discomfort. Consult with a healthcare provider to determine the most suitable pain management plan.

2. *Exercise and Physical Therapy: Regular, low-impact exercise is crucial for maintaining joint flexibility and strength. Physical therapy can provide targeted exercises to improve joint function and alleviate pain.

3. Weight Management: Maintaining a healthy weight reduces the stress on weight-bearing joints, like the knees and hips. Weight loss can significantly relieve symptoms and slow disease progression.

4. **Assistive Devices:** Depending on the affected joints, using assistive devices like braces, canes, or orthotic insoles can provide additional support and relieve joint strain.

5. **Joint Protection:** Employ proper joint protection techniques during daily activities. This includes being mindful of posture, avoiding overuse, and using ergonomic aids when necessary.

6. **Balanced Nutrition:** A well-balanced diet rich in nutrients supports joint health. Omega-3 fatty acids, found in fish and certain seeds, can help reduce inflammation.

7. **Emotional Support:** Dealing with chronic pain can take a toll on mental health. Seeking support from friends, family, or a therapist can help individuals cope with the emotional challenges of osteoarthritis.

8. **Surgical Options:** In some cases, surgery may be necessary. Individuals should explore surgical

interventions like joint replacement in consultation with their healthcare provider.

9. **Lifestyle Adaptations:** Adjusting daily routines and living spaces to accommodate mobility challenges is important. Simple changes, such as installing handrails or modifying the home environment, can make a big difference.

10. **Stay Informed:** Being educated about osteoarthritis can empower individuals to make informed decisions about their treatment and self-care.

Coping with osteoarthritis is an ongoing process, and a multidisciplinary approach involving healthcare professionals, physical therapists, and mental health experts can provide valuable support. Customized management plans that consider the individual's unique circumstances are essential for effectively dealing with the challenges posed by this chronic joint condition.

Lifestyle Tips for Managing Symptoms

Living with osteoarthritis can be challenging, but certain lifestyle adjustments can significantly help manage symptoms and improve your quality of life. Here are some essential tips for effectively managing osteoarthritis:

1. **Regular Exercise:** Incorporate low-impact exercises into your daily routine to strengthen the muscles around affected joints and improve joint flexibility. Activities like swimming, walking, and cycling are gentle on the joints and can help reduce pain and stiffness.

2. **Weight Management:** Maintaining a healthy weight is crucial for managing osteoarthritis. Excess weight puts extra stress on weight-bearing joints, exacerbating symptoms. A balanced diet and weight loss, if necessary, can alleviate discomfort.

3. **Physical Therapy:** Consult with a physical therapist to learn exercises and techniques tailored to

your specific needs. Physical therapy can improve joint function, alleviate pain, and enhance mobility.

4. **Pain Management:** Discuss pain management strategies with your healthcare provider. Over-the-counter or prescription pain relievers, topical treatments, and heat or cold therapy can help manage pain and inflammation.

5. **Joint Protection:** Be mindful of your joint health in daily activities. Practice good posture, avoid overexertion, and use assistive devices like braces or orthotic insoles when needed.

6. **Balanced Nutrition:** A diet rich in vitamins, minerals, and omega-3 fatty acids can support joint health and reduce inflammation. Consult a dietitian for personalized dietary recommendations.

7. **Rest and Relaxation:** Adequate rest and sleep are essential for managing osteoarthritis. Listen to your body and allow it to recover between activities to avoid overuse injuries.

8. **Stress Reduction:** Stress can exacerbate pain and inflammation. Incorporate stress-reduction techniques like meditation, deep breathing, and mindfulness into your daily routine.

9. **Adaptive Tools:** Use adaptive tools and devices to simplify daily tasks. Tools like jar openers, reachers, and specially designed utensils can make life with osteoarthritis more manageable.

10. **Footwear and Orthotics:** Choose comfortable, supportive footwear and consider custom orthotic insoles to help distribute pressure evenly across your feet and reduce joint strain.

11. **Hydration:** Staying well-hydrated is important for maintaining joint function and supporting overall health.

12. **Emotional Support:** Seek support from friends, family, or support groups to cope with the emotional challenges of living with a chronic condition.

Remember that effective management of osteoarthritis often involves a combination of these lifestyle tips. It's important to work closely with your healthcare team to create a personalized management plan that addresses your unique needs and circumstances. By implementing these lifestyle changes, you can take control of your osteoarthritis symptoms and enjoy a better quality of life.

Chapter 12

Current Research and Future Directions

Osteoarthritis (OA) is a widespread, degenerative joint disease that affects millions of individuals worldwide. It is characterized by the progressive deterioration of joint cartilage, leading to pain, stiffness, and reduced mobility. While several treatments and management strategies exist, ongoing research is essential to improve our understanding of the disease and develop more effective interventions. Here, we'll explore some of the current research areas and potential future directions in the field of osteoarthritis.

Early Detection and Diagnosis:

Current Research: Early diagnosis of OA is crucial for initiating timely intervention. Researchers are exploring advanced imaging techniques, such as magnetic resonance imaging (MRI) and biochemical markers, to detect cartilage damage at its earliest stages.

Future Directions: The development of non-invasive biomarkers and point-of-care diagnostic tools may lead to more efficient early detection and diagnosis of OA.

. Disease Mechanisms:

Current Research: Scientists are investigating the underlying molecular and cellular mechanisms that drive cartilage degradation and inflammation in OA. Research is uncovering the roles of various factors, including cytokines, enzymes, and genetic predispositions.

Future Directions: A deeper understanding of OA's pathophysiology may lead to the development of targeted therapies that can modify the disease progression and provide better pain relief.

Current Research: Stem cell therapy and tissue engineering approaches are being explored to regenerate damaged cartilage. Researchers are investigating the use of various cell types and scaffolds to encourage cartilage repair.

Future Directions: Developing safe and effective regenerative treatments for OA remains a priority. This includes optimizing cell sources, delivery methods, and understanding the long-term outcomes of these therapies.

Disease-Modifying Osteoarthritis Drugs (DMOADs):

Current Research: The search for DMOADs continues, with researchers investigating potential drug candidates that can slow down the progression of OA and modify the underlying disease processes.

Future Directions: Identifying and developing safe and efficacious DMOADs remains a major goal in OA research, as these drugs have the potential to reduce the need for surgical interventions.

. Personalized Medicine:

Current Research: Advances in genomics and proteomics are allowing for more personalized approaches to OA treatment. Understanding an individual's genetic and molecular profile can help tailor treatment plans.

Future Directions: The integration of personalized medicine into OA management could lead to more precise and effective interventions, potentially reducing adverse effects and improving outcomes.

Biomechanics and Joint Protection:

Current Research: Researchers are studying joint biomechanics and the effects of various interventions like braces, shoe modifications, and orthotics on OA symptoms and progression.

Future Directions: Optimizing joint protection strategies through biomechanical research and designing innovative devices to reduce joint stress is an area with significant potential.

Lifestyle Interventions:

Current Research: Studies are ongoing to determine the most effective lifestyle interventions, such as exercise programs, dietary modifications, and weight management, for managing OA.

Future Directions: Future research may uncover novel lifestyle interventions and further refine existing strategies for improved OA management.

Telemedicine and Digital Health:

Current Research: The use of telemedicine and digital health tools to deliver OA care is gaining traction, especially in remote or underserved areas.

Future Directions: Continued development of digital health platforms and tele-rehabilitation programs can enhance access to care and support patients in self-management.

Multidisciplinary Care:

Current Research: Studies are exploring the benefits of a multidisciplinary approach, involving healthcare providers from various specialties, in managing OA patients.

Future Directions: Establishing guidelines and models for effective multidisciplinary care, along with improving the coordination of care, can lead to better patient outcomes.

Patient-Reported Outcomes and Quality of Life:

Current Research: Researchers are increasingly focusing on assessing the impact of OA on patients' quality of life and overall well-being.

Future Directions: Future research may prioritize the development of patient-reported outcome measures that encompass the holistic experience of living with OA, helping guide treatment decisions.

In conclusion, the field of osteoarthritis research is dynamic and continually evolving. Ongoing studies are shedding light on the complex mechanisms of the disease, with the aim of developing more effective treatments and management strategies. The future holds promise for earlier detection, regenerative therapies, personalized medicine, and innovative interventions, all of which may lead to improved outcomes and a higher quality of life for individuals living with osteoarthritis. As researchers continue to make breakthroughs, the future of OA management looks increasingly hopeful.

The search for innovative and effective therapies for osteoarthritis (OA) is ongoing, with several promising approaches on the horizon. These emerging therapies aim to provide improved pain relief, slow disease progression, and enhance the overall quality of life for OA patients.

Biologics and Disease-Modifying Osteoarthritis Drugs (DMOADs):

Biologics, such as growth factors, stem cells, and platelet-rich plasma (PRP), are being explored for their potential to stimulate cartilage repair and reduce inflammation. DMOADs, which can modify the disease course, are a particularly exciting area of research. These drugs aim to slow OA progression and delay the need for surgical interventions.

Gene Therapy:

Gene therapy holds promise for OA by targeting specific genes responsible for cartilage degradation and inflammation. This approach seeks to modify gene expression to protect cartilage and promote repair.

Nanotechnology:

Researchers are investigating the use of nanotechnology to develop drug delivery systems that can specifically target OA-affected joints. These nanocarriers can enhance the effectiveness of medications while minimizing systemic side effects.

Tissue Engineering and 3D Printing:

Tissue engineering techniques, including the use of 3D-printed scaffolds and biomaterials, offer the potential to create replacement cartilage and bone structures. These engineered tissues can be implanted to restore joint function.

Neurostimulation:

Neurostimulation therapies, such as spinal cord stimulation and peripheral nerve stimulation, are being explored to manage OA-related pain. By targeting nerve pathways, these treatments can provide pain relief in a localized and targeted manner.

.

Exosome-Based Therapies:

Exosomes, small vesicles secreted by cells, are being investigated for their regenerative potential. Exosome-based therapies may offer a novel approach to stimulate cartilage repair and reduce inflammation in OA joints.

immunomodulatory Agents:

Agents that modulate the immune response, such as anti-IL-1 and anti-TNF drugs, are being studied for their potential to reduce inflammation in OA. These drugs aim to mitigate the inflammatory cascade associated with the disease.

AI and Machine Learning:

Artificial intelligence and machine learning are being used to analyze patient data, imaging, and biomarkers to better predict OA progression, tailor treatment plans, and improve overall patient care.

Innovative Surgical Techniques:

Advances in minimally invasive surgical techniques, such as robotic-assisted joint surgeries, are improving the precision and outcomes of joint replacement surgeries for OA patients.

These emerging therapies represent a promising shift in the management of osteoarthritis. While many of these approaches are still in the experimental or investigational stage, they hold the potential to provide more effective, targeted, and less invasive treatments for OA in the future. As research continues to progress, these therapies may offer new hope for individuals living with this chronic joint condition.

Chapter 13

The Impact of Osteoarthritis

Osteoarthritis (OA) is a chronic joint condition that can have a profound impact on affected individuals, their families, and society as a whole. This degenerative disease, which primarily affects weight-bearing joints such as the knees, hips, and hands, presents several significant consequences:

1. **Pain and Discomfort: One of the most noticeable impacts of OA is the persistent pain and discomfort it brings. Individuals with OA often experience pain that limits their ability to perform daily activities, affecting their overall quality of life.

2. **Reduced Mobility:** OA can lead to stiffness and reduced joint mobility, making it challenging for individuals to walk, climb stairs, or engage in physical activities. This loss of mobility can lead to decreased independence.

3. **Emotional and Psychological Effects:** Living with chronic pain and physical limitations can take a toll on mental health. Many OA patients experience depression, anxiety, and a reduced sense of well-being.

4. **Financial Burden:** OA imposes a substantial economic burden on individuals and healthcare systems. Costs associated with medical treatments, medications, assistive devices, and, in some cases, surgery can be significant.

5. **Impact on Work and Productivity:** OA can affect an individual's ability to work and be productive. Many individuals with OA may require workplace accommodations or even early retirement due to their condition.

6. **Reduced Quality of Life:** OA has a profound impact on an individual's overall quality of life. It can limit social interactions, hinder participation in hobbies and recreational activities, and lead to feelings of isolation.

7. **Increased Risk of Comorbidities:** OA is often associated with comorbid conditions such as cardiovascular diseases, diabetes, and obesity. These

comorbidities further impact a person's health and well-being.

8. **Caregiver and Family Burden:** The burden of OA extends to caregivers and family members who often take on additional responsibilities to support affected individuals.

9. **Healthcare Resource Utilization:** OA is a major driver of healthcare resource utilization, from primary care visits to specialist consultations, imaging studies, and surgical procedures.

10. **Societal Impact:**

On a broader scale, OA presents a societal impact in terms of healthcare costs, lost productivity, and the need for improved infrastructure and accessibility to accommodate individuals with mobility challenges.

Recognizing the substantial impact of OA highlights the importance of ongoing research and the development of more effective treatment strategies. Early diagnosis, targeted interventions, and a comprehensive approach to managing OA can help mitigate the physical, emotional, and economic burden this condition places on individuals and society. Additionally, raising awareness about OA can promote understanding and empathy, ultimately leading to better support and improved outcomes for those affected by this chronic joint disease.

Hope for Improved Treatments

The future of osteoarthritis (OA) management holds promise, with ongoing research and advancements offering hope for more effective treatments. Here are some reasons to be optimistic about the future of OA care:

1. **Regenerative Therapies:**

Emerging regenerative therapies, such as stem cell treatments and tissue engineering, show great potential for repairing damaged cartilage and slowing disease progression. These therapies aim to regenerate joint tissues, providing lasting relief and improving joint function.

2. **Disease-Modifying Drugs:**

The development of disease-modifying osteoarthritis drugs (DMOADs) is a focus of research. These drugs have the potential to alter the course of the disease, reducing pain and the need for surgical interventions.

3. **Personalized Medicine:** Advances in genomics and personalized medicine are leading to more targeted and effective treatments. Tailoring interventions to an individual's unique genetic and molecular profile can enhance outcomes and reduce side effects.

4 **Innovative Surgical Techniques:**

Minimally invasive surgical techniques and robotic-assisted joint surgeries are becoming more refined. These approaches offer improved precision and shorter recovery times, enhancing the patient experience.

5. **Advanced Pain Management:**

Researchers are exploring novel pain management strategies, including neurostimulation techniques, to provide targeted relief for OA-related pain.

6. **Biological Therapies:**

 Biologic agents, such as growth factors and monoclonal antibodies, are being investigated for their potential to reduce inflammation and promote joint health in OA.

7. **Digital Health Solutions:**

Telemedicine, wearable devices, and digital health platforms are enhancing access to care and supporting patients in self-management, providing more options for OA management.

8. **Comprehensive Care Models:** The development of comprehensive and multidisciplinary care models can lead to more effective and patient-centered OA management.

The commitment of researchers and healthcare professionals to improving OA care is driving the development of innovative treatments and approaches. While some of these treatments are still in the experimental or investigational stage, they hold the potential to transform the way OA is managed, offering individuals living with OA hope for a future with less pain, improved joint function, and an enhanced quality of life. As research continues to progress, there is reason to believe that the landscape of OA treatment will continue to evolve, providing new and more effective options for those affected by this chronic joint condition.

Living with Osteoarthritis

Living with Osteoarthritis (OA) can be a challenging journey, but with the right strategies and support, individuals can still lead fulfilling lives. Here are some key aspects of living with OA:

1. **Pain Management:** Managing chronic pain is often a central focus for individuals with OA. This can involve medications, physical therapy, and lifestyle

modifications to minimize discomfort and improve daily functioning.

2. **Mobility and Exercise:** Maintaining joint mobility and muscle strength is crucial. Low-impact exercises, such as swimming and gentle stretching, can help improve mobility and reduce pain.

3. **Weight Management:** For those with OA, maintaining a healthy weight is essential. Excess weight places added stress on joints, exacerbating symptoms.

4. **Joint Protection:** Learning how to protect your joints during daily activities is important. Proper ergonomics, assistive devices, and pacing yourself can reduce strain on affected joints.

5. **Emotional Well-Being:** Living with OA can be emotionally challenging. Many individuals experience depression and anxiety. Seeking support from friends, family, or mental health professionals is essential.

6. **Adaptive Tools:** Using adaptive tools and devices can make daily tasks easier. These can include jar openers, grabbers, and orthotic insoles.

7. **Healthy Nutrition:** A balanced diet rich in nutrients supports joint health and overall well-being. Omega-3 fatty acids found in fish have anti-inflammatory properties that can help reduce joint inflammation.

8. **Sleep and Rest:** Adequate rest and quality sleep are important for OA management. Ensuring a comfortable sleeping environment and managing pain can improve sleep quality.

9. **Regular Monitoring:** Regular check-ups with healthcare providers help monitor OA progression and ensure that the treatment plan remains effective.

10. **Living Life to the Fullest:** Despite the challenges, many individuals with OA find ways to adapt and continue pursuing their passions and interests. Finding joy in hobbies, spending time with loved ones, and maintaining an active social life can enhance overall quality of life.

Living with OA requires resilience, adaptability, and a commitment to self-care. By actively engaging in pain management, exercise, and lifestyle adjustments, individuals with OA can regain control over their lives and continue to enjoy a meaningful and fulfilling existence. While OA presents its unique set of challenges, it does not define a person's identity or limit their capacity to lead a rewarding life.